SURVIVING A WORLD PANDEMIC

Well-being and Survival in a World Pandemic

Dr Megan

Little Black Book of Survival: Series 1

CONTENTS

The 10 step guide

Preface

"Even the darkest night will end, and the sun will rise" - Les Misérables

In 2020 most of the world is in lockdown due to a new World Pandemic- Covid -19. This new virus sweeping the globe is the novel coronavirus. Some experts suggest that there were clues as early as Spring 2019 that a World Pandemic was on its way. There have been many previous Pandemics . The common theme has been that these have been respiratory viruses that were highly contagious, spread rapidly and caused widespread death. Deaths from Pandemics have been well in excess of the total of all the wars in history which puts the threat to you in perspective . In order to survive you need a military style drill operation in your household to combat this virus. Don't panic , but you have to act quickly, methodically and early to increase the chance of you and your family surviving this pandemic.

This is the first book in the Little Black Book Series of surviving difficult situations in your life. We will take you through a short guide to surviving a world pandemic. This short guide will give you a ten step plan for surviving a pandemic , protecting your physical health, mental health, and finances.

My sincere thanks and love to my family and friends and in particular to my beautiful mother Sophia who has taught me love, strength and compassion all my life.

STEP 1 HOW DO I PREPARE FOR A PANDEMIC?

Prepare and prevent , do not repair and repent.

The World Health Organisation defines a Pandemic as a worldwide epidemic crossing international boundaries that is:

1. able to infect humans
2. able to cause disease in humans
3. able to spread from human to human

A virus is an ultra-microscopic (20 to 300 nm in diameter), metabolically inert, infectious agent that replicates only within the cells of living hosts, mainly bacteria, plants, and animals: composed of an RNA or DNA core, a protein coat, and, in more complex types, a surrounding envelope. There are 1.5 million viruses in wildlife. A virus that jumps from animal to human is called Zoonotic. The virus can then mutate, jump from a human back to another animal and back to another human. There is no treatment or vaccination currently for Covid-19 - the novel coronavirus. These viruses cause panic and death. The SARS virus in 2002 was a new coronavirus and affected 23 countries with 8000 people affected. The same again with MERS in 2012 affected 27 countries and there were 858 deaths. Viruses hijack the host body in order to replicate quickly and take over all organs. Coronavirus 19 can live on hard surfaces for days which makes public places a real health hazard. Look out for those early warning shots ! Pandemics presents us all with many challenges as we adjust to a new way of living. The worst case scenario is a rapidly spreading highly contagious respiratory virus that kills on average 1 in 3 people. There is much uncertainty and this is the start of potentially a long period of adjustment in all our lives. Essential facilities will be impacted when their workers become potentially infected and are unable to work. What will happen during a lockdown? You will need to provide food, water and electricity for your family for a period potentially up to four months . You will also need financial cover to pay for all your bills for the same amount of time.

What is a lockdown or a Quarantine? Well the term Quarantine originates from Italy in 1600 from the word quarantina, which is a variant of Upper Italian (Venetian) meaning a period of isolation of forty days. It originated from the Black Death.

Remaining in lockdown is the most vital early measure we can actively take in our lives. I instigated my own lockdown three weeks prior to the official government lockdown having watched updates from China, Korea and Australia. Always look at the patterns of previous pandemics . Don't forget that the Spanish Flu had three waves of deaths with the second one being far more deadly than the first one.

Remember other factors influence the lifting of lockdowns. Don't be a casualty of a political decision. Do not be lulled into a false sense of security. In the midst of a pandemic the governor of Georgia in the United States of America opened beauty salons, tattoo parlours and other non- essential businesses. Now the sceptics would say that if businesses are forced to stay open then they can no longer claim on their insurance policies. In a way the government forces the hand of businesses to "open".

Germany suffered triple daily rates of coronavirus when they eased the lockdown in May 2020. The same thing happened with Italy when they lifted the lockdown in Lombardy, and Japan and China .

I would strongly advise against going out during the lockdown lifting of restrictions. More likely than not, lifting lockdown will be an economic decision made by the politicians of your government. Stay vigilant and watch disease and death trends in your area like a stockbroker watches his shares and stocks.

Give yourself two to three weeks to come to terms with quarantine or lockdown / stay at home orders. Your productivity and morale will be very low in the first few weeks of a lockdown- this is entirely normal.

This will be a short 10 step guide to surviving a pandemic and establishing a routine that optimises your physical and mental health and wellbeing.

Embrace this golden opportunity of a world pandemic to recalibrate your life. Distill all your values down to the core important elements of your life. This is the time to embrace change and prove your warrior spirit and survive this pandemic. You must be ready for a coming crisis. Your life and the lives of your loved ones will depend on it. Be your own hero in this crisis.

Stay Prepared....

Stay ready so you won't have to get ready. In an ideal world you would be ready and prepared for a pandemic at all times. You should be. But what does this involve? First and foremost always ensure that you have at least three months supply of essential medicines and prescriptions. An emergency medical pack is an essential part of your preparation. Countries that are prone to hurricanes and tornados often give advice to their citizens in relation to preparing an emergency pack.

Include the following items in your **<u>emergency home kit:</u>**

Epipen (if you have allergies)
Paracetamol
Aspirin low dose 75mg and high dose 300mg
Antibiotics (preferably a penicillin)
Hydrocortisone cream
Hydrogen Peroxide 6% solution
Steroid cream
Ear drops
Antibiotic and Refreshing Eye drops
Anti-histamines
Anti-diarrhoeals
Fluid/electrolyte rehydration
Anti-sickness tablets
Cough syrup
Nasal saline spray
High dose Vitamin C tablets
High dose Vitamin D dose
Zinc
Birth Control
Face masks- suggest N-95 as well as FP3 respirator masks

First Aid Kit
Steristrips
Skin glue
Micropore tape
Steristrips
Bandages
Swabs
Tourniquet
Rubbing alcohol
Box of latex or non-latex gloves
Electronic blood pressure machine
Oxygen Saturation Measurement Device

Oxygen Concentration machine, nasal cannula and masks

General items
Matches
Water filter jug 3L with additional filters
Bottled water to last four months

I am a strong advocate of face masks and I would strongly recommend purchasing a FP3 respirator mask from a hardware store with some extra filters . These last about three months with each new filter generally. They cost around £15. The outside and inside of masks can be cleaned with alcohol wipes after each use .

It is vital to have a small oxygen concentrator at home . They weigh on average between eight and twelve kilograms. They take atmospheric air and concentrate oxygen to produce high concentration and high flow oxygen. They cost between £1000 to £2000 but are a worthwhile investment. There is a short three step installation that takes on average fifteen minutes . It is also wise to have a method of measuring oxygen saturation in blood, whether this be through a small saturation machine or a phone app that allows fingertip oxygen concentration measurement.

If you have a car it's worthwhile investing in a digital tyre inflator to have in your car. They cost around £30 and along with your emergency jump leads form a very useful basic car first aid kit. Try to turn your car engine on once a week and drive and reverse the car forward and backwards for a minimum of fifteen minutes a week.

What if I need to go to hospital ?

Keep a fully stocked emergency hospital bag in your room. Include one weeks supply of your medication and a print out of your prescription. Also include items of personal protective equipment such as gloves, masks and gowns. Take electronic copies of all your health records on your phone including all recent clinic letters and blood results. Keep a hard copy of your clinic letters in this emergency bag to take with you if you need to go to hospital. Keep an extra mobile phone charger and a paper copy of your emergency contacts in your emergency bag. The common emergencies will be discussed further in Step 5 How to Stay Alive.

Stay One Step Ahead

In a world pandemic stay ahead of the news by watching news from as many sources as you can. If Italy had watched the news about China closely during the Covid-19 pandemic start in January 2020, there were valuable lessons to learn from the Chinese lockdown in Wuhan as well as early social distancing and mask utilisation. Likewise the United Kingdom did not heed the advice of the Chinese , Italian or Spanish which led ultimately to a very high death rate and a late lockdown. Be proactive in seeking out international news, not only to acquire more information about other countries ahead of yours on the pandemic curve but also about your own country.

Watching countries ahead of you on the curve can also enable you to make decisions about anticipated resource shortages. For instance the Australian media showed toilet paper, antibacterial products and flour shortages well in advance of these shortages in the United Kingdom. The media in your own country can shield you about some aspects of shortages , population spread and deaths in order not to create panic. For instance in the U.K. there was a shortage of Covid-19 tests and people that clearly had died from Covid without a positive test we're not included in the death statistics. The United Kingdom also initially excluded all Covid patients in nursing homes that died, underestimating the daily death rate by more than 5000 cases. I personally found the Australia and Chinese news broadcasts straight and to the point upon which I was able to make effective decisions about early lockdown. In fact I advised my family and friends to go into voluntary lockdown three weeks before the official lockdown .

Food shopping

You need an efficient system for food shopping. Register online as soon as possible with all the supermarkets. In the United Kingdom you will find on average three supermarkets in your area that will deliver. Anticipate the challenges early and book your online delivery slots as soon as possible and a few weeks apart . These slots go very early so be aware. There are some apps now available to enable you to identify available slots. In the first few weeks of the pandemic in the United Kingdom it was near impossible to get an online delivery slot. You can try calling the supermarket customer services phone line to book a vulnerable delivery slot if you fit the criteria. Also try food wholesalers that supply restaurants they may have a surplus of ingredients due to restaurants being closed under lockdown conditions. Failing that, one younger member of the family ideally one with no underlying health problems should be nominated for this duty. That individual should try to make the least number of trips possible until online delivery can be restored. They need to wear either a hazmat style suit or a hoodie with the hair covered , glasses or goggles, an airtight mask - long sleeves and long trousers. Take three pairs of thick latex gloves and take some alcohol antiseptic wipes. If you are going by car , wear the full suit upon leaving your house and don't touch anything until you reach your car. Don the full "personal protective equipment" . Your car essentially becomes a "dirty area". Once inside your car , wipe your gloves down with one antibacterial wipe and your steering wheel. Start the car and aim to get to the supermarket 10 mins prior to opening. Avoid large branches or superstores. The exposure is too high , the number of employees is high and surviving is a game of Russian roulette. Don't make your odds any higher than you need to. Take a plastic freezer bag which will be your "dirty bag" you take instore with your mobile phone , an extra pair of gloves , your car keys and alcohol wipes inside. The inside will be "clean" theoretically . Leave a clean freezer bag in your car for your return .

Park in the drop off zone or short stay part of the supermarket parking. The name of the game is : minimising risk. Keep two large floor antibacterial wipes in your hand . Clean the handles of your trolley and base with your antibacterial wipe. Take one clean supermarket bag that you have brought from home and lay in the bottom of your trolley. Try to avoid produce from hotspots for Coronavirus. During Italy's worsening crisis I tried to avoid fresh fruit or vegetables from Italy however it's quite difficult in some cases ascertaining the country of origin of items. Although nutritionally beneficial try to avoid items like broccoli or cauliflower that are difficult to thoroughly clean.

Over the counter medicines such as Paracetamol, Vitamin C and Vitamin D were in short supply in the United Kingdom, you need some useful strategies. Call ahead of time and find out expected delivery times from shops and pharmacies and time your visit accordingly. Purchase from small pharmacies or large pharmacies at ten minutes before the morning opening times . This may be at seven or eight in the morning . Phone your local store ahead of time . In some small branches of supermarkets it may be possible to reserve some items with the manager ahead of time . I generally found early on Monday mornings the best time to get the most stock in. My local supermarket had deliveries at 1am.

Stock up items for a minimum of three to four months. Food wholesalers may be the best option if you are having difficulty getting key items. When you have finished your shopping, load all the items into your car in a designated "dirty zone " lay a sheet on the bottom of your car boot in preparation. After you have finished loading the shopping into your car, dispose of only your gloves and the used shopping bag that was under your shopping into a bin. Use your alcohol wipes immediately to both hands for more than 20 seconds . I suggest using two of these. Transfer your items inside your freezer bag into the clean freezer bag. Clean and disinfect hands again . Open your car and sit down. Put fresh gloves on and drive home in your mask and full protective gear. Coronavirus and highly infectious respiratory viruses stay in the air for several hours and may be transferred from your clothing. You need a strict protocol within your house to disinfect your shopping. I suggest you divide your apartment or house into clean and dirty zones. The area just inside your front door is the designated dirty area . Further back will be the "clean area" as will the rest of your house. As far as respiratory viruses such as SARS-COV2 coronavirus they can be killed with antibacterial/ alcohol based disinfection and also at temperatures above 20 degrees Celsius.

Take your shopping to the dirty zone designated in your house and leave one bag for "dirty items". Take the gloves off (they have been outside the house) and dispose. Put on the third set of gloves and start cleaning all the items and move them from the dirty to clean zone in your house Leave the "dirty" bags in the "dirty" zone which should be at the entrance area of your house or apartment. Leave a large clean box in the clean zone . Using your mask, gloves , goggles and long sleeved clothes and take each item and wipe with a fresh antibacterial wipe and place the clean item into the clean zone. Discard the anti-bacterial wipe. For bread or other bagged items remove the bag and decant into clean freezer bags with a no touch technique . With fruit and vegetables place them into a large basin to be washed later with warm water and Milton baby sterilising fluid and soak for thirty minutes . Then thoroughly wash each item before placing in your fridge. Be extremely careful with the freezer as respiratory viruses thrive in cold temperatures. Disinfecting your shopping will take approximately an hour. After all items have been added to the clean box, wipe your gloves with an antibacterial wipe. Wash hands throughly with hot water and soap . Then take your mask off. If it is a FP3 respirator mask then you need it clean the outside of the mask with an alcohol wipe. Make sure the inside is cleaned well and the straps. Clean your goggles with a disinfect-ant wipe. If it is a disposable mask take it off and discard in a large bin bag with all the used alcohol wipes. Lastly strip off all your dirty clothes into another black bin bag. Empty the clothes from the black bin bag into the machine without touching the items and wash on a hot cycle above 60 degrees Celsius. Head straight to the shower for a hot bath including washing your hair well.

Stock up on the staples as early as possible in the Pandemic . Use all the freezer space you have for fish, meat and other high protein items. You can vacuum pack these so they don't take up a lot of space . Use two of your freezer drawers for these items. Use your other two drawers for frozen fruit , berries, and vegetables . The majority of your stock should be pasta, rice, lentils , canned to-matoes and other pulses.

I would consider buying an additional fridge freezer or a deep chest freezer. You can freeze milk and bread in the spare freezer.

A large part of the anxiety associated with pandemics is the uncertainty of the timescale. Take control of the situation and make sure you have enough core stock items to keep you going for at least six months in the worse case scenario. You will find by taking control of several small steps in emergency planning during the pandemic your anxiety levels will be lowered. Dedicate one spare room or area in your apartement ot house to stock for the pandemic. Keep all like items in one place or shelf together. Arrange the items in chronological date order depending on expiration date . Put the items that are due to expire in front . Use five empty bookshelves to organise by category.

STEP 2 WHAT SHOULD I EAT?

In the midst of a pandemic try to exclusively cook homemade food from fresh ingredients to minimise infection risk. Good homemade food will boost your immune system and mood. Try not to turn to or rely on delivery, comfort or convenience foods. If you are overweight or diabetic you will already know these are major risk factors for death from Coronavirus Covid-19. Have regular meals , and stick to regular meal times. Choose healthy options such as fruit, a small handful of unsalted nuts and seeds for snacking.

Eat five portions of fruit and vegetables a day to make sure you're getting a range of vitamins and minerals.

It is vital to take a daily supplement of Vitamin D after consultation with your doctor. It is usual for this to be recommended mainly in the winter months but with lockdown it is worthwhile taking this every day alongside your high dose Vitamin C and Zinc supplements. There is some anecdotal evidence that a low vitamin D level worsens outcomes in coronavirus.

Zinc is a mineral that's essential for good health which is required for the functions of over 300 enzymes involved in many important processes in your body. Your body doesn't store zinc, so you need to eat enough every day to ensure you're meeting your daily requirements. Stress, inflammatory foods, and low activity can increase chronic inflammation. This can impair your immune system from fighting infections. Several food groups are anti-inflammatory in nature. As Hippocrates said "let good by thy medicine and medicine thy food".

The Pandemic Diet

Specific foods with the highest anti-inflammatory properties are the following:

Berries
Berries are packed with fibre, vitamins, and minerals. Try to include strawberries, blueberries, raspberries, and blackberries in your diet. They are post potent in their raw form. Berries also include anti-oxidants called anthocyanins. Anthocyanins have anti- inflammatory effects that may reduce your risk of disease. Blueberries increase the number of your natural killer cells that are the frontline of your immune system.

Fatty Fish
Perhaps one of the best sources of proteins and long chain omega-3 fatty acids EPA and DHA. The best types of fish are salmon, sardines, herring, mackerel and anchovies for their anti-inflammatory effect. They also significantly improve your mood.

Shellfish
Shellfish contains high levels of zinc and are a low calorie option. Mussels, Oysters, Crab and shrimp are also high sources of zinc. These should be eaten with caution in pregnancy.

Green Leafy Vegetables
Green vegetables and avocados are a great food staple. They are packed with potassium , magnesium, fibre, carotenoids, and tocopherols.

Green tea
Green tea contains epigallocatechin-3-gallate (EGCG). EGCG stops inflammation by reducing pro-inflammatory cytokine production and damage to fatty acids in your cells.

Manuka honey

Try to incorporate one tablespoon into your daily diet. The anti-bacterial, antimicrobial, anti-inflammatory and antiviral nature of Manuka honey can boost your immune system and even improve your gut health

Onions

Onions contain antioxidants and compounds that fight inflammation, decrease triglycerides and reduce cholesterol levels . Their potent anti-inflammatory properties may also help reduce high blood pressure and protect against blood clots. Onions and leeks belong to a family of superfoods known as the allium family. Garlic, onions, leeks and chives have potent health-enhancing qualities. Onions contain calcium, potassium, vitamin C and folate.

Garlic

Garlic has been used by humans for thousands of years and was used in Ancient Egypt for both culinary purposes and its health and therapeutic benefits. There are many documented health benefits . Garlic has documented benefits to the cardiovascular , lungs, and immune system. Try to include at least 4 cloves a day in your diet.

Apple Cider Vinegar

This is vinegar made from fermented apples . There is some evidence for its antibacterial effects and it can help in control of diabetes by lowering blood sugar . Try to include a spoonful as a salad dressing or diluted in a glass of orange juice .

Nuts

In order to increase your zinc levels try eating nuts such as pine nuts, peanuts, cashews and almonds . Nuts also contain other healthy nutrients, including healthy fats and fiber, as well as a number of other vitamins and minerals. Cashews have one of the highest levels of zinc of any of the nut group. Use them as snacks during the day in small portions as they have been linked to a reduction in risk factors for some diseases, like heart disease, cancer and diabetes.

Pulses

Pulses like beans , lentils and chickpeas are also good sources of zinc all contain substantial amounts of zinc. However these are less well absorbed than meat products. Meat is also an excellent source of zinc. The highest amount of zinc is found in red meat. However all types of meat do contain zinc. They can however have an inflammatory effect so reduce consumption to 2-3 times a week.

Seeds

Seeds are a healthy addition to your diet and can help increase your zinc intake. The highest zinc contents are in pumpkin seeds, sesame seeds and squash seeds. They not only boost your zinc intake but contain fibre, healthy fats, vitamins and minerals complimenting your balanced diet. They can also reduce your cholesterol and blood pressure.

Dairy

Cheese, yoghurt and milk provide a host of nutrients, including zinc. They have high amounts of bioavailable zinc, meaning maximum absorption by your body. Dairy also has vital protein, calcium and vitamin D to boost your immunity.

Eggs

Eggs should be a staple part of your pandemic diet. They contain a moderate amount of zinc and can help you meet your daily target. Their is an abundance of vital nutrients in eggs such as proteins, B vitamins, selenium and choline which are vital for cell repair.

Whole Grains

Whole grains like wheat, quinoa, rice and oats contain some zinc. You need to be aware that they also include phytates, which can bind to zinc and reduce its absorption .Whole grains contain more phytates than refined versions and will likely provide less zinc. However, they are considerably better for you and a good source of many important nutrients like fibre, B vitamins, magnesium, iron, phosphorus, manganese and selenium. Whole grains can provide a source of zinc in your diet. However bear in mind the zinc they provide may not be absorbed as well as other sources due to the presence of phytates.

Potatoes

Both regular and sweet varieties of potatoes contain no fat, sodium or cholesterol. Equipped with almost half your daily value of vitamin C, high potassium, vitamin B6, magnesium and antioxidants you should make this a staple of your pandemic diet.

Dark Chocolate

Finally some good news! Include dark chocolate into your pandemic diet. Brimmed full of iron, magnesium and zinc in some ways it is a superfood. Chocolate comes from cacao, which is a plant with high levels of minerals and antioxidants. Commercial milk chocolate contains cocoa butter, sugar, milk, and small quantities of cacao. In contrast, dark chocolate has much larger amounts of cacao and less sugar than milk chocolate.

The best way to ensure you are getting enough is to eat a varied diet with good sources of zinc, such as meat, seafood, nuts, seeds, legumes and dairy. These foods can be easy and delicious additions to your diet.

Mindful eating

When you devour your meal on autopilot while engrossed by your surroundings - the conversation , mobile phone , television, or computer you do not appreciate the sumptuous taste and aroma of your meal. You're also less likely to feel content because you have missed the act of eating. Don't multitask whilst eating. Focus your full attention on the meal at hand.

Hydration

With respiratory viruses it is essential to consume large amounts of hot drinks every hour to two hours. Generally speaking these virus are killed at high temperatures . They can reside in your nose and throat for up to 6-8 hours before spreading to the lungs .You need to get a saline nasal spray and use this three times a day. I find Sterimar the best brand to use. Gargle with hot salty water three times a day to keep any virus particles in your throat at bay. Try to drink between 8-9 glasses of water during the day. When exercising you will need a bit more hydration. Try to have your caffeine early in the day and no later than 2pm for a restful nights sleep. Excess caffeine can also lead to increased irritability and anxiety levels during this time . Try not to turn to alcohol or recreational drugs as coping strategies during this time. We will discuss other strategies for coping.

STEP 3 HOW DO I STAY FIT IN QUARANTINE?

"I hated every minute of training. But I said don't quit. Suffer now and live the rest of your life as a champion" Muhammad Ali

Most gyms will be closed during lockdown. Even when they open , bear in mind they are going to be a hotbed of bacteria. There is no filtered air systems in gyms currently, therefore for respiratory viruses it's a disaster. It's similar to being in a plane for 2-3 hours. Therefore it is worth investing in some basic gym equipment at home . Ideally you want to restrict the cost of this to around £100. An exercise bike, rowing machine and some free weights and a skipping rope should make up the basics of your "home gym". Try to dedicate a room or area for your gym equipment . Try to start with around twenty minutes of cardio exercise a day and vary this depending on the day to avoid boredom. Do not go outside for exercise during a pandemic. With joggers nearby and an increased respiratory rate one can see how virus particles can be generated and spread on a larger scale and at a faster rate. Exercise is essentially a high risk aerosol generating procedure and I personally feel the risks of cardio exercise outside in a busy metropolitan area is high risk. Obesity is a major risk factor for Covid-19 so it is essential to measure calories carefully based on your height and age and your target weight.

Online workouts

There are a large number of online workouts you can access for free on YouTube and Instagram. Access High Intensity Training , Barre, Yoga, Pilates or Boxing circuit workouts. Make sure your exercise regime is a combination of cardio exercise as well as strength training with weights. You can also incorporate yoga and Pilates workouts into your weekly regime. Give yourself 1-2 days off a week depending on how you are progressing. Exercise is crucial in managing anxiety and stress levels. If you are working from home try to get up and move every hour.

The most popular online workouts seem to be:

F45
This popular network provides live zoom classes about 3 times a day and if you miss any workouts you can access any time.

Core Collective
This is a luxury London based studio that has launched online fitness streaming classes. These include yoga, pilates, high intensity training, and strength training.

ROWBOTS
ROWBOTS is a British Rowing Rowing workout co-founded by the footballer, Gareth Bale, combining floor and rowing based workouts that focus on strengthening the body and mind. They've adapted workouts and created some live body weight/floor-based HIIT workouts daily.

The Body Coach
Joe Wicks is broadcasting live workouts on his Instagram which are available for 24 hours from first posting and uploaded on his Youtube channel. His P.E inspired classes are a great way for kids to stay fit whilst off and parents too.

Shreddy

Due to an increased demand for more home workouts, fitness app Shreddy has created a free 14-day challenge via their Instagram to help their community keep fit and active whilst at home. There are shared workouts listed in their weekly timetables. Some of these will be shared on their Instagram feed.

Bounce

Trampolining studio Bounce has launched taster sessions for free and reduced the price of its trampolines.

Base PT HIIT Workouts

Base PT is an app which give you a virtual workout. On the app you have access to the live 1-2-1 sessions with top personal trainers. These workouts are perfect for anybody looking to improve their fitness. The 30 minute high-intensity sessions can be at your 'base' of choice - whether that be from your lounge, loft or local park.

1Rebel

1Rebel have launched an app service whilst their gyms are shut due to Coronavirus. They will have their iconic Reshape and Rumble workouts available online.

Centr

Centr is an app that has been developed by celebrity Chris Hemsworth and his wife, Elsa Pataky.They offer a free six-week trial. The app is a personalised, digital health and fitness platform which features a team of renowned experts hand-picked from the worlds of fitness, nutrition and mindfulness. The workouts are primarily HIIT-focused and require little to no gym equipment, ideal for quarantine.

BLOK

Whilst their studios are shut across the UK, BLOK has now developed BLOKtv - a series of live streamed classes in partnership with Beats by Dr. Dre on Instagram Live.

STEP 4 HOW DO I PROTECT MY MENTAL HEALTH?

"It is during our darkest moments that we must focus to see the light" Anon

The first few weeks into a Pandemic you will be feeling very strong emotions and it is important to acknowledge these and most importantly be easy on yourself . Once you have taken control of organising your quarantine space and supplies as described above, you need to give yourself some time for mental rest and recuperation. Embrace and fee; each emotion you have to the maximum . If you are upset - let the tears out and cry. You will feel better afterwards. Do not suppress any of the emotions you will feel during quarantine or the pandemic. Some of the feelings you will experience early on will be sadness, denial, anxiety and shock. Your productivity and morale will be at an all time low. Do not expect too much from yourself in the early days. Anxiety stems mainly from uncertainty and lack of control. Take control of the things you can, to lower your anxiety levels. You cannot control the lockdown or the quarantine period- the virus controls that. You can control how you deal with the challenges of the pandemic. First of all, be gentle with yourself. This is an unprecedented sudden change of all the things you hold of value . Your world is about to be turned upside down. You will survive this, like you have survived many challenges in the past. Use your warrior spirit.

If you have pre-existing mental health issues, low mood or suicidal thoughts you need to contact your medical team urgently as you will need more personalised tailored care.

What is Depression?

Depression is a distressing experience. Physical symptoms of low mood affect the way that we think, what we do and how we feel. It can then spiral into a vicious cycle, making it harder to cope, and live our everyday lives. Negativity of our thoughts become unhelpful and ob-structive. The vicious cycle continues with low mood and apathy. Even-tually this impacts on our physical and mental health. Everything may seem worse through the prism of depression , particularly a world pandemic. It will be difficult to see any positivity in your situation. Depression can make us critical of ourselves unfairly. It is important to make a major distinction between your thoughts and feelings and actual facts. You may feel apprehensive and bad about your situation but that does not mean your life is all bad. You might think that your feelings equate to facts. They don't . You may feel quite hopeless about the future ,which usually is a temporary feeling. Research has shown that depression can also stem from your genetics, your chem-ical imbalances, challenging life experiences, and ongoing difficulties. The causes may be different but the symptoms are very common to all. Research suggests low serotonin (a chemical) within the brain, apathy and negative thoughts all lead to depression. It may be difficult to carry out the activities of daily living when you are depressed. If these thoughts become unmanageable and/or you feel suicidal please see medical help urgently. Cognitive Behavioural Therapy may help with your treatment. It is common to feel depressed and anxious in the midst of a pandemic.

What is Anxiety?

Anxiety is a normal emotion, which although unpleasant does not cause harm. In your everyday life you may feel nervous, jittery, your heart pounding, fast breathing, sweating, trembling, dizziness and a feeling of dread. Anxiety is useful in warning you and protecting you from danger. Your body responds using the Fight or Flight response. This is a primal response from our caveman days to allow us to run away from dinosaurs! This includes quickened breathing enabling more oxygen to get to our organs and muscles and an increased heart rate to increase blood flow to our muscles in preparation for "flight". All other non urgent bodily processes slow down, such as saliva production and digestion . When the danger is over, the body returns to normal. When anxiety becomes a chronic problem you may perceive danger in situations when they are not. Your thought process is stimulated in the same fight or flight pathway with all the resulting symptoms. This can exacerbate your anxiety further. This is all too common in a pandemic. You are in an unknown situation , the news and media are telling us about the daily deaths and individuals grief stories from around the world. Your thought process will be configured along the negative pathway and worse case scenario - "catastrophising events". Picture your worrying thoughts as if they were trains at the station. You watch them go past you as you stand on the platform. You do not get on the train with your thoughts and you certainly do not go down the tunnel chasing one of your worries. Usually in anxiety when there is a trigger, you can choose to avoid that situation and that does form part of the treatment of anxiety disorders. In those situations you may begin to limit your daily activities to avoid those stressors and that may impact your life . However in a pandemic we are being told to restrict our daily activities, self-isolate, and quarantine. We are told of the ever increasing death rate in our city and country. You are not able to easily avoid the trigger. You can however restrict your time watching the news or reading media which is very helpful.

Techniques to try

Focus on what is good about isolating at home. It can be something as small as the ability to sleep in , or having the time to reconnect with old friends that you haven't talked to in years. Maybe it's having the ability to try out new hobbies or getting unexpected enjoyment out of different activities. What activities can you spend time on that you couldn't before? Discovering what your silver lining is, can help you refocus your time and energy positively. Worrying is unhelpful when the control is not in your hands. This may because these are future events which have yet to occur, over which you have no control. Will your country enforce mandatory vaccination for Covid-19? Will you able to go on holiday as planned in July? Will you lose the money for your holiday? You don't know, and you cannot control it. If it happens everyone will have to deal with the same contentious issues not just you. You are not alone. Try to eliminate worry about uncertain events, unpredictable events which you cannot control. This takes away all the pleasure from your current life, albeit in a pandemic there may not be much pleasure! You cannot control your family's safety in a pandemic, but you can reduce risk by instigating a family lockdown to avoid external exposure to the virus. We will discuss some concrete techniques to help lower our anxiety levels. The Hertfordshire NHS Trust has some very useful online documents and information to assist in this which has been discussed and will be shown below.

Keep a Worry Log

If any concerns or worries come into your mind , write them down in details in your worry log. If it is an immediate worry such as an unpaid bill then action it there and then if you can. Worries are either present, past or future.

Schedule a worry appointment

Schedule a worry appointment in the evening around 8pm for approximately 30-40 mins to start with. You are taking control by allocating a set time to list and address your concerns. This time allocation may need to be longer in the beginning and take this into account when planning. As your technique improves you may be able to reduce this time period. Don't do anything else in your worrying time apart from worrying. Find a nice quiet area where no-one will disturb you. Try not to do this immediately before bedtime.

Any time a worry pops into your mind, write it down in the diary shown below. Slowly you will recognise any unhelpful patterns that are contributing to your anxiety, you can make changes to replace these with new ones that reduce anxiety and improve your coping skills. A common pattern is making every thought into a catastrophe. Cognitive Behavioural Therapy can help you identify this and provide you with methods to overcome these. Refocus on the present time and enjoying the details within your surroundings. Keep repeating this process to reconfigure your worry pathway. In your allotted time you can worry as much as you want and address each worry in turn. The strength of some of the worries may have diminished. Worries seem to be time-sensitive and decrease in their potency with the passage of time. Be strict about your worry appointment and any new worries that come to mind will have to be included in the next day's worry diary.

Worry Diary

Date and Time	Situation	Your Worry (e.g. 'What if')	How anxious do you feel on a 0-10 scale?	Classify Your Worry (either Hypothetical or Practical)	
				Hypothetical	Practical

Photo from the Wellbeing Services, Hertfordshire Partnership University NHS Foundation Trust

Barriers or blocks and possible solutions

Barriers or Blocks	Solutions
I don't know if it's a hypothetical or practical worry	Use the chart. Really consider if there is anything you can do about it right now
I can't refocus	It takes time, keep practicing. Use your senses
I'm worrying what if I worry.	Use the technique, this is a hypothetical worry.
I can't stop worrying at the end of worry time	Plan in an activity after worry time so you have something to refocus on.

Once you have written down your worry, and written in the columns above, refocus on the present moment. Focus on what is going on around you and tune your attention to it. It is harder to worry when you are really focused in the moment. Consider your five senses and focus on those. Focus on the present moment and take in the details of your room - the textures of your curtains and the patterns, the decorations on your window sill, the colour scheme of your bed, and the texture of the fabrics. Open your window and absorb the smells. I live in London and this part isn't too pleasant! Do not consider this technique as distraction. It's merely focusing on the present time and whether that is the smell of the plants and trees in your garden, the smell of your lunch, the taste of the vegetables you are munching on or the small details of the objects around you it recalibrates you. Writing down all your new and old worries focuses on documenting your concerns and helps the recalibration. Any time a worry pops into your mind, write it down and then recalibrate into the present. Refocus on the present time and enjoying the details within your surroundings. Keep repeating this process to reconfigure the worry pathway.

Meditation

Meditation has several documented benefits. It can boost morale and productivity as well as increased energy, peace and joy. Start by dedicating 10 minutes a day to meditation. Even starting with short sessions will reap immense benefits. Slow and deep breathing is the way to begin making each last for 5 seconds. This will help reduce your anxiety levels and help you reset. Sometimes we are so lost in our thoughts that we are missing everyday life. There are several great meditation apps and youtube videos available which I would recommend. Headspace, Calm and Insight Meditation apps are amongst the top rated apps.

Avoidance of stressors

Strictly limit your news intake to twice a day for 15-20 mins each time. Do not stay on social media all day streaming continuous updates. You do need accurate information, but a long stream of this will ultimately lead to an increase in stress and anxiety. Set boundaries for yourself on how often you'll watch or read coronavirus news each day. Review your column of worry in your diary to see common stressors. You will need to work through these with Cognitive Behavioural Therapy.

Cognitive Behavioural Therapy

Cognitive Behavioural Therapy is a structured psychological treatment which recognises that the way we think (cognition) and act (behaviour) affects the way we feel. CBT is a method of focussed and realistic problem-solving. Many people with anxiety actively avoid situations that are stressors. CBT helps you confront your fears and approach challenges in a practical manner. A range of techniques may be employed. You can actively learn the difference between productive and unproductive worries, letting go of worries and solving problems. Relaxation, breathing techniques, muscle relaxation, and other methods of controlling anxiety and the physical symptoms of tension can be mastered.

Access to CBT

CBT involves working with your therapist and identifying regular thought and behaviour patterns that are increasing your anxiety. Therapy can be delivered one-on-one with a therapist, in groups, or online. CBT is often combined with behavioural therapy. Things that are out of your control can accentuate our anxiety and subsequently other mental health issues.

Situation	Emotion	Automatic thoughts (images)	Evidence for	Evidence against	Alternative thought	Rate Emotion again
Who with? What doing? Where?	What did you feel? (one word) How intense? (0-100%)	What is going through my mind? What is the worst thing that can happen? What does it mean about me if it is true?		Am I jumping to any conclusions that are not justified by the evidence?		(0-100%)

Mindfulness

Your senses - touch, taste, smell, sight and sound are your portal into the present space. But when you are lost in thought, your thoughts rob you of the present time. Your senses are picking up your environment but your thoughts overpower your senses. There are so many beautiful but basic sights around you everyday. When you are making your morning coffee, stop and soak up the beautiful scent. The early morning smell from your open window is priceless. The beauty and diversity of flowers in your neighbourhood. One of my neighbours makes an amazing casserole once a week - envisage the mouth-watering aroma of the fried spices and roasted chicken smell! Notice how your dress or clothes feel and look against your body. Enjoy the freshblinen smell of your bed sheets and the feel of your bed in the morning. Enjoy the comforting touch of your loved ones. Embrace the sensation of water and bath foam on you during your shower. Make an effort to carry out your daily tasks with maximum effort, attention and love. It will make a significant difference to your life. Rest between your actions. Resist the urge to multitask. Putting full stops between actions in your day, can move the focus onto each and every task. This will ground and relax you, provide clarity to your consciousness and refresh your energy levels.

Children

There are whole books dedicated to this subject which are worthwhile exploring. Remember how hard this is for you, and how confusing and scary it must be for a child who may not fully understand what is happening. Children need adults to be positive role models to navigate these choppy waters. Take time to ask your children how they are feeling and remain approachable so that they feel the channels of communication are open. They will be missing their friends, school and their relatives as well. Let them know if they feel upset or sad you will always be there. Play regularly, paint, enjoy music and do sports together.

Stay in the Moment

Listen earnestly. The majority of us listen to about 15 % of what people are telling us. We are usually too busy planning what to say next, analysing what they are saying, or losing interest after a few seconds. Actively try and make it your intention to fully listen to what the other person is saying to you, without distraction. Be natural about your response when it's your turn to speak. As we have discussed you are not equal to your thoughts. You are merely the observer of your thoughts. Separate this concept of your thoughts and your identity. Disconnect from them and observe objectively.

Take back control of the situation

Some days will be better than others. Whether you are working from home or not it is important to establish a routine that works for you. It is essential to design a structure to your day. Try to sleep and wake up around the same time every day. Aim for a sleep period of around 8-9 hours avoiding daytime naps. Have a pen and paper or worry diary next to the bed. You can then write down anything making you feel anxious, so it can be dealt with the next day. Make sure your bedroom is dark, quiet, cool and that your mattress is comfy. Avoid having clocks on display near your bed. If you can manage a 15 minute stretch or light exercise in the morning before your breakfast do that. At a minimum you need twenty minutes of cardio exercise a day and twenty minutes of weight training. Schedule in lunch breaks and tea/coffee breaks regularly and stay well hydrated aiming for 6-8 large cups of water a day. The lockdown in the United Kingdom allowed for daily outdoor exercise. Exercise helps reduce anxiety and stress and it's a vital part of your quarantine routine. If you live somewhere quieter than a capital city then time in nature or parks is a relaxing way to do your outdoor exercise . Observe all the small details of your walk outside including the cloud patterns, the details on the leaves and the types of trees and birds surrounding you. Feel the sunshine on your skin and absorb the smells of the outdoors. If you are indoors consider cultivating your houseplants and indoor herbs. In your anxiety diary note down a list of friends and family that make you feel happy, joyful and relaxed. On another page note down the acquaintances , friends and family that make you feel bad. Hard as it may be, for the period of the lockdown and quarantine period try to stay away from contact in your second list. Stay connected to all those who are on your first page. Call them regularly and arrange video calls. If you are living in quarantine with people that aggravate you at times, try to minimise contact whereby possible . In optimal times that can be challenging but in the times of a pandemic nerves are on their edge and adding this further conflict to the mix can fray your nerves even more. Establish boundaries both geographically and emotionally with those individuals. However for most people you will be quarantined with your loved ones and this is an ideal time to reconnect, talk and enjoy activities together in the home. Take a moment to pause, take a deep breath, and appreciate that you are alive in this very minute. This minute is your life.

STEP 5 HOW DO I STAY ALIVE?

Within each pandemic each virus will have its own set of signs and symptoms. In 2020 the Pandemic was Covid-19 so we will discuss this in a little more detail. The disease is mainly passed on from droplets in breaths, coughs, laughs and sneezes. It can live on hard surfaces for 72 hours. It can take 2-20 days before signs and symptoms appear.

Signs and symptoms of Covid-19

Loss of taste and smell
Temperature
Cough
Abdominal pain
Diarrhoea

Skin changes - painful red nodules, hives
Headache
Visual Disturbances
Sore throat
Chest pain
Shortness of breath
Dizziness
Intense tiredness
Other non specific signs

Surveillance

Aim to measure your oxygen level, pulse rate, respiratory rate and temperature twice daily. You can install an app on your phone to measure your oxygen saturation level. I use the Oximeter app. You need to have an oxygen level ideally above 97% on room air. Covid-19 can act in some ways like carbon monoxide poisoning whereby your oxygen level falls to a low level with very few early symptoms. If you find your oxygen reading is low take a few deep breaths and try again with a different finger. If it is still low this is of concern and you need to seek medical advice. With coronvirus you can have low oxygen saturations with very few other symptoms.

Measure the number of breaths you take in one minute . Try to breathe as you would normally breathe. The normal rate is 12-18. If it is higher than this it indicates you are struggling to breathe. This is a warning sign.

Your temperature should be lower than 37 degree Celsius ideally. If any of these parameters are outwith normal you need to seek early medical attention.

Do not take a negative Covid-19 test as gospel, they have yet to mass produce a highly sensitive test for Covid-19.

It is understandable that in the midst of a pandemic you may try to avoid any routine hospital or clinic or dental visits . Any hospital exposure can risk catching this deadly virus . Recent research has shown that

20% of patients caught Covid-19 when they were in hospital for another reason.

During the Covid-19 pandemic, hospitals in Belfast Northern Ireland divided all the Covid positive patients to the Belfast City Hospital and tested patients and instigated quarantine and self isolation for those undergoing urgent cancer treatment in the other hospitals . Particularly impressive is how they managed to continue performing kidney transplants during a world pandemic.

Unfortunately other emergency conditions such as strokes, heart attacks, and appendicitis can still happen at times of pandemics. Try to identify local hospitals that are "clean" and which have been identified as Covid-19 hospitals to seek help.

Common medical emergencies

These urgent conditions amongst others need urgent medical care, delay can cause permanent damage and death.

Toothache : there may a number of causes such a dental abscess, fractured filling, or cavity. There may be nerve irritation. Contact your dentist immediately. If you cannot get hold of your dentist then most large hospitals have a maxillofacial department that you can contact and be seen as an emergency patient. In addition if you cannot open your jaw, have a temperature, eye swelling it's vital that you are seen in the emergency setting. Simple measures are eating soft food, regular mouthwash with warm saline washes, painkillers, and penicillin antibiotic emergency dose can be temporising measures A hairdryer or hot towel on the affected side can provide temporary relief.

Appendicitis: this can starts with vague pain around the belly button, you may be off your food, feel mild nausea. In approximately 24-48 hours it may localise to your right lower abdominal area with associated vomiting. This is surgical emergency and you need to attend the emergency department.

Bowel Obstruction: this can start with abdominal pain, nausea, vomiting, failure to pass wind and failure to open your bowels. This is surgical emergency and you need to attend the emergency department.

Heart attack: this may present in a number of different ways in women and men. It may cause nausea, shortness of breath and general malaise in diabetics who may have "silent' heart attacks. It can cause chest tightness centrally moving to the jaw or left side of the arm with associated tingling. It may be associated with shortness of breath. It needs emergency medical treatment. If you anticipate delays then taking a 300mg aspirin tablet is prudent (as long as there are no contraindications).

Stroke: a stroke is a serious life-threatening medical condition that happens when the blood supply to part of the brain is blocked. The brain needs the oxygen and nutrients provided by blood to function properly. If the supply of blood is restricted or stopped, brain cells begin to die. This can lead to brain injury, and death.
There are 2 main causes of strokes:
ischaemic – in 85% of cases where the blood supply is stopped because of a blood clot
haemorrhagic – where a weakened blood vessel supplying the brain bursts.
Mini Strokes are transient ischaemic attacks (TIA), where the blood supply to the brain is temporarily interrupted. It can last a few minutes or persist up to 24 hours.
Strokes are a medical emergency and urgent treatment is essential. The sooner a person receives treatment for a stroke, the less damage is likely to happen.
The main symptoms of stroke can be remembered with the word FAST:
Face – the face may have dropped on one side, the person may not be able to smile, or their mouth or eye may have dropped.
Arms – the person with suspected stroke may not be able to lift

both arms and keep them there because of weakness. Speech – their speech may be slurred or the person may not be able to talk at all despite appearing to be awake; they may also have problems understanding what you're saying to them.

Time – Act early and call an ambulance

Aneurysms: An aneurysm is the enlargement of an artery caused by weakness in the arterial wall. Often there are no symptoms, but a ruptured aneurysm can lead to fatal complications. Most aneurysms do not show symptoms and are not dangerous. However, at their most severe stage, some can rupture, leading to life-threatening internal bleeding.

Aneurysms affect a variety of arteries. The most significant aneurysms affect the arteries supplying the brain and the heart. An aortic aneurysm affects the body's main artery.

The rupture of an aneurysm causes internal bleeding.

The risk of an aneurysm developing and rupturing varies between individuals. Smoking and high blood pressure are major risk factors for the development of an aneurysm.

Some types of aneurysm may need surgical treatment to prevent rupture. Doctors will only operate on others if they are life-threatening. Seek urgent medical attention.

Visual loss: Vision loss is caused by problems at any point along the visual pathway from the eyes to the brain, and sudden vision loss is an emergency. Vision involves light passing into the eye and being transformed into electrical signals that are processed in the brain. Light enters the eye through an opening called the pupil and is changed into electrical signals by cells located toward the back of the eye in the retina. These signals then travel from the eyes through the optic nerves to the brain. In the brain, the occipital lobes process the visual information to make sense of it. Problems at any point along this visual pathway can cause vision loss. This can occur over a period of a few seconds or minutes to a few days. Vision may become blurry or cloudy, completely absent, or affected by flashing lights or specks in the visual field called floaters. Part of the field of vision or the entire field of vision may be affected. It is helpful to cover one eye and then the other to determine whether one eye or both eyes are affected. Sudden vision loss is most often painless but may be associated with eye pain, redness, and headache. Any sudden change in vision is potentially serious, even if it involves only part of the visual field or resolves on its own. Common causes include eye trauma, blockage of blood flow to or from the retina (retinal artery occlusion or retinal vein occlusion), and pulling of the retina away from its usual position at the back of the eye (retinal detachment). Inflammation of the blood vessels that supply the eye and the optic nerve or inflammation of the optic nerve itself can also cause vision loss. A sudden blockage of blood flow to the occipital lobe of the brain (as can occur with a stroke) is another common cause of sudden vision loss.

Renal failure: Sometimes kidneys are no longer able to filter and clean blood. This can cause unsafe levels of waste products to build up. This is known as kidney (or renal) failure. Unless it is treated, this can cause death. Healthy kidneys clean waste products from the blood by making urine. They also balance the amount of certain elements in your blood (such as sodium, potassium, and calcium), and make hormones that control blood pressure and red blood cells.
Kidney (renal) failure is when kidneys don't work as well as they should. The term "kidney failure" covers a lot of problems. It may be related to diabetes, high blood pressure, glomerulonephritis or polycystic kidney disease. Your kidney may be blocked by a kidney stone or scar tissue causing severe pain.

Signs to look out for:

loss of appetite
nausea
vomiting
swelling of the hands, feet and face (oedema)
internal bleeding
confusion
seizures

coma
abnormal blood and urine tests
high blood pressure
shortness of breath
chest pains
numbness and tingling
easy bruising
itching
fatigue
headaches
muscle twitches and cramps

Fractured or dislocated bones: usually as a result of an injury. They need urgent medical attention.

Burns: Burns and scalds are damage to the skin usually caused by heat. You need immediate first aid with cold running water to the area. Wrap the burn in cling film and keep the patient warm and well hydrated. Seek urgent medical advice.

Spreading skin infections/Necrotising fasciitis: skin infections can start as small red inflamed areas from a break in the skin or an abscess. They occur more frequently in diabetics or immunocompromised people. They can proceed and spread rapidly. Seek urgent medical advice.

GI bleed: losing blood from any cavity - it can be either vomiting fresh blood, coffee ground vomit - digested blood, or passing blood from your bowel. Seek urgent medical advice.

Critical ischaemia of a Acute limb ischaemia occurs when there is a sudden lack of blood flow or blockage to a limb. It can be caused by a clot/embolism or thrombosis, or rarely by dissection or trauma. This is surgical emergency and can lead to the loss of your limb. It is highly treatable. Delayed treatment (beyond 6 to 12 hours) can result in permanent disability, amputation, and/or death.Symptoms of acute limb ischaemia include:

Pain
Pale leg
Numbness
Coldness
Pulselessness
Paralysis

Deep Vein Thrombosis/Pulmonary Embolus: Deep vein thrombosis (DVT) is a blood clot that develops within a deep vein in the body, usually in the leg. Blood clots that develop in a vein are also known as venous thrombosis.
They usually occur in the larger vein that runs through the muscles of the calf and the thigh. It can also occur in the pelvis or abdomen.It can cause pain and swelling in the leg and may lead to complications such as clots in the lungs /pulmonary embolism which can lead to death.

STEP 6 FINANCIAL SURVIVAL

"Save money and it will save you" Anon

How can you save yourself from financial destruction during a Pandemic? Reading about the plummeting economy and the loss of jobs is enough to panic all of us. The headlines about Covid-19 and reports of how it will impact the economy and potentially lead to a recession are all a cause for concern. We will not be able to appreciate the full impact of the quarantine and lockdown on many businesses for the time being. As with everything, the amount of planning that you do prior to a situation is critical to your survival. The aim is for this to be minor glitch in your long term plans rather than a life-changing crisis.

Early Survey

Make an early assessment whether your job will survive the pandemic or not. Keep your options open and be ready to pivot employment. If you are self-employed make assessments as to whether your business is likely to stay open and whether you can afford to keep your employees on. Consider a part-time remote based job using some of your skills as bridging employment.

Furlough Scheme

If a company is unable to operate or they have no work for staff to do during the pandemic, workers are put on "furlough". This means that they are kept on the payroll and not made redundant. Contact your employer to arrange this directly.

Check your Contract

Dig out the copy of your employment contract and read it in detail. Make sure you think about how that might need to be worked out between you and your employer. If you need to shield how will your employer support you? Many employers are creating flexible working patterns in light of the pandemic . Ask what they can do to help you out. Carefully review your benefits. My advice is not to leave your children in nursery or school during a pandemic. Look carefully at your sickness benefits at work - in anticipation of getting sick for a pro-longed period of time: Confirm if your employer offers paid sick or family leave. Review your other company benefits and speak to your colleagues.

Contact your Human Resources Department to make sure you are aware of all that is on offer. In addition, your state might offer un-employment insurance benefits during this period. If you have any pri-vate insurance plans check all the terms and conditions to see whether your mortgage payments may be covered during this time.

Early Planning

It is important to keep calm and make a honest assessment of your situation so you can make any urgent adjustments as necessary. Can-cel all unecessary direct debits and subscriptions. If you don't already have an emergency bank account create one online with your bank.
You need to survive for 3 – 6 months with your emergency savings account. The specific amount you set aside will depend on your per-

sonal circumstances. The money should be easily accessible. Ideally you will have been making regular direct debit deposits to your emergency savings account.

Crisis Budget

Immediately adjust your lifestyle and implement the crisis budget. Appropriate planning for your crisis budget will ascertain how much is in your account and how long that will last you if you are off work for 6 months. This will decrease your anxiety levels as it introduces a level of certainty to your situation. You can either use a spending app to track your expenses or a paper template. Have printouts of your statements and work out the basic monthly outgoings and income. This emergency budget eliminates any non-essential spending enabling you to prepare adequately for the essentials like food, and accomodation. Knowing how much you need to survive will help prevent panic because you know exactly what to cut back on. You will be living off a fixed spending plan. If there is a deficit you may need to top up your budget with a home based job. There will be many pandemic-related short term jobs that you can apply to. The salary may not be as high as your "normal' job but hopefully your spending will not be as high during a pandemic either. If you are renting then speak to the landord about having a month or two "rent holiday" or "deferment'. If you have a mortgage ask for a 3 month "mortgage holiday". Cancel any direct debits that are not necessary such as gym memberships, and deliveroo that you won't be using.

The Future

We don't know how long this economic recession will last and how long recovery will take. Your crisis budget may need to stay in place for a year or more.

Don't make any rash decisions about selling or buying assets or investments during this time. Take good financial advice and if you can afford to diversfy stocks and shares. Stay focussed on the big picture and long term goals. No matter how adequate your emergency savings are, you never know how long you might need to cover expenses in the event of a loss of income. Try to find new income streams during this time. After the pandemic you might be tempted to go back to your prior spending habits, but you mustn't - you need to rebuild your stock of emergency savings. Remain on your crisis budget until you have recuperated your funds.

No one's financial situation is guaranteed, so we all mustplan for unforeseen circumstances.

STEP 7 INTERACTING WITH OTHER PEOPLE

The most dangerous time in a pandemic is when the lockdown is lifted. Many of us in recent weeks have begun working remotely from home, if we haven't been furloughed or laid off. Universities and schools have cancelled classes and people have stopped using public transport with a domino effect restaurants, shops, bars, and gyms have shut. Major events were cancelled in all countries and in America at least 42 states had enforced stay-at-home directives. Social distancing, health authorities argue, can dramatically slow the rate at which the infection spreads, helping to ease the burden on the health care system. When many countries were in lockdown with strict stay-at-home orders and lockdowns in place, many decisions about avoiding the risk of getting the coronavirus were simple. There was no option of eating out, people didn't have to think about whether dining in a restaurant is safe if the restaurant was closed. Around the worldwide lifting of lockdown is occurring mostly prematurely, with low levels of precautions in place. The onus is on you to weigh up your risks on your own.

The decision will not be easy. There is a lot of contradictory information out there, and it can be a maze to navigate. Choose your own sources of reputable information and use them as a guide. Personally I rate the leaders of Ireland and New Zealand very highly indeed. Ireland's Taoiseach Leo Varadkar himself a physician made some very sensible decisions during Ireland's lockdown as did Jacinda Ardern and

I kept a close eye on both of these leaders as a guide. Let's look closer at the spread of respiratory viruses and in particular Covid-19 so we can make a decision about whether to venture outside again.

Spreading of the Virus

The vital process of contact tracing has enabled us to find "super-spreaders", where one person ends up infecting tens of others. Through deductions we can identify and highlight the key risk factors that create infections. Covid-19 spreads by droplets that exit from people's mouths and noses during laughing, sneezing, coughing, breathing and talking. Other unaffected people breathe in the virus droplets in the air that can stay for around 15-20 minutes. Contrary to the 2m or 6 feet arbitrary distance, Covid-19 virus particles can actually travel 20 feet and sometimes more depending on the wind speed. This makes sense if we think about smelling someone's cigarette smoke from across the street. Each breath from a Covid-19 positive person releases approximately 100 droplets concentrated with the virus. These can land on surfaces, stay in the air, or get inhaled by a passer-by. The virus can also get into your system through your eyes, nose, or mouth. That's the main risk, and that's why face masks are essential. I found it extremely annoying that due to lack of face masks worldwide , various governments changed their early advice and were advocating not using any. Staying home as much as possible, even if you believe you aren't infected can slow the infection rate known as "flattening the curve", but most of all protect you from new infection.

Taxis and Public Transport

If you do need to use such a service, don't use one during a pandemic. Remember that contaminated hands pose a risk to drivers and riders, so if it is an emergency and you need to use one take precautions. Use full PPE as described previously . Scrupulous hand hygiene, washing or sanitizing your hands before getting in the car/train and not touching your face at all. Open a window during the journey and face the window.

Schools and Children

In Ireland, public health officials are encouraging a very sensible "no parties, no playdates, no playground" policy. In most epidemics and pandemics young children are the transmitters. Children can spread the disease, and at least a small risk of severe illness is present for all age groups including a potentially fatal Kawasaki-type syndrome that can cause ITU admission. It is very responsible to shut down schools. Several hundred children interacting in close quarters is very high risk. It does have a political and economic impact on their parent's jobs and employment hence the push from governments to force school openings. The risk of under-reaction is much more catastrophic than the risks of over-reaction.

Restaurants

If restaurants in your area re-open in coming weeks, or if they remain open be very careful. Think about the surfaces you touch, the table, menu, cutlery, sauces and the transmission from your waiter or waitress. How often can you sanitise your hands in a restaurant setting. Who is cooking your food? Have they been exposed to Covid-19? Proceed with extreme caution.

The Human Touch

While social distancing does mean physical separation from coworkers, friends and family, it doesn't mean being socially cut off from them. Technology makes it easier than ever to reach out to loved ones across the world. While a video chat isn't quite the same as physically seeing or hugging someone, it can be a worthwhile substitute during this difficult time. Maintain a connection with people you care about whether that's via phone calls, video chats, emails, and texts. Having this social outlet can remind you that you're not alone, even if you're physically by yourself.

STEP 8 QUARANTINE FATIGUE

> *"Our fatigue is often caused not by work, but by worry, frustration and resentment."* Dale Carnegie

At the moment we have no indication of the length of our quarantine period or social distancing recommendation. It may last up to one more year . Hopefully you will have established a routine. Remain flexible and able to adapt to new challenges.

Maintain your routine

Find out what routine is best for you in your structure of your day. Waking up too early means you are tired for the rest of the day. Sleeping in too late leaves you sluggish and unproductive for the rest of the day. Pick the sweet time which will usually be 30-45 mins later than your previous alarm clock time. Establish whether you perform better doing your daily exercise in the morning or afternoon , and before or after meals. Introduce new recipes for your meals and evaluate whether you need to cut calories or increase them in this next phase of "lockdown".

Self-care

Decide whether you need more or less personal time away from your family in the house or apartment. Maintaining time away from other family members is vital in self-preservation during quarantine . During this uncertain and stressful time we may feel more fatigued than usual and this is entirely normal. Some families will be working from home as well as home schooling which can be a real challenge. Each individual may respond differently to the stressors that quarantine presents. There may be a real sense of longing for friends and family that you haven't seen for a few months. Video chats and zoom can help but for some this is not enough. The biggest challenge is the lack of a change of environment. When the lockdown has eased you may consider doing one hour walks early in the morning to minimise your risk of exposure to others . This is particularly hard in London. Maintaining a rigorous 20 minute cardio workout daily will improve your mood significantly and ease any anxiety. It will also help you sleep better at night. Taking care of your health is also a helpful form of self-care, can reduce your stress and boost your immune system. This involves things like eating healthy meals (lots of fruits, vegetables and whole grains), making sure you're getting exercise and also getting enough sleep. One worrying feature of the lockdown was the massive increase in alcohol sales. It's important to keep this in check as you may feel vulnerable during this situation and it may be easy to turn to alcohol during this time. It is not an effective long term method of controlling your mood.

The pandemic and social distancing guidelines have introduced novel opportunities to connect with colleagues and friends and family. Use each day to check in with friends and loved ones. Try to contact with three friends or family each day to check in and provide support.

Try to be kind to yourself and lenient during this time. Use your best dishes to serve up lunch and dinner and make it a memorable event . Dress well when at home as if you would be going out to work or to meet friends. Get lost in the flow of doing things you love. Utilise self care and self love. This is different for everyone. It may be soaking in a bath with candles and music. It may be having a nice dinner with your nice plates and glasses, playing your favourite song on the piano, snuggling with your dog or using your rowing machine. This is the time for your guilty pleasures and treating yourself whichever way makes you happy and content. We love doing these things so much that we often lose ourselves in them. Our love and attention is focussed in the present moment and this overshadows our anxieties. Incorporate more enjoyable flow activities in your weekly routine, and your happiness will catapult. Make a list of your favourite activities and try one of them each day. Make a list of your all time favourite songs for each from the age of 12 onwards. Then play one favourite song from each year of your life each day.

Consider a short youtube based meditation for 10-20 minutes each evening. You will overcome this , you are strong and have overcome many challenges before in your life. Keep the faith in your strength. Life will go on.

STEP 9 TREATMENT OF A PANDEMIC

There is currently no vaccine and no treatment for Covid-19. My advice is don't become a guinea pig. In 2006 an independent drugs trial at Northwick Park Hospital ended in disaster. Healthy young volunteers were recruited to trial a new drug called THN1412. This caused multiple organ failure in six of the volunteers. This was concluded to be "unpredicted biological action of the drug in humans". The drug was being trialled for treatment if leukaemia and auto-immune conditions.

Treatment of SARS

The SARS vaccine was a huge failure. It caused fatal lung infections in the animals during the animal trials. To date there has never been a successful vaccine for any of the viruses of the coronavirus family. Dr Fauci a world expert in immunology alluded to the theory of "vaccine enhancement". This is where the vaccine makes you worse when exposed to the actual pathogen. At the time of publication early human trials are taking place in Oxford for the Covid-19 vaccine.

Treatment of the Ebola virus

There is no treatment for Ebola. Early treatment is advocated with providing fluids and electrolytes intravenously and early oxygen treatment . The Food and Drug Adminstration has not licensed any drugs for Ebola treatment. In 2018 two trial treatments, called regeneron (REGN-EB3) and mAb114 were used in the Democratic Rpeublic of Congo which showed overall survival was much higher. These two antiviral drugs currently remain in trial use for patients with confirmed Ebola.

This guide is how to survive a Pandemic. My advice is not to volunteer for an unknown vaccine or drug trial if you want to survive this pandemic.

Covid-19 Convalescent plasma trials

There are now trials to treat COVID-19 using the blood plasma from those who have already recovered from the illness have begun. I haven't seen any evidence to support this and I don't advocate treatments with no evidence to support them.

Oxygen treatment

From my own reading of international colleagues accounts and early evidence of Covid-19 I can draw some similarities between Covid-19 and carbon monoxide poisoning and altitude sickness. Does Covid-19 causes an increase in endogenous carbon monoxide poisoning in the body? We know that Covid-19 causes very low oxygen levels over a long period of time. Your red blood cells carry oxygen from your lungs to all your organs and the rest of your body. Red blood cells do this through haemoglobin, which is a protein consisting of four "haemes". Haemes have a special kind of iron ion, which is very toxic in its free form, but it is safe in its packaged bound form. The iron ion can be carried around safely by the haemoglobin and used to bind to oxygen when it gets to your lungs. The virus binds to the haem part of your haemoglobin molecule in your red blood cells. When you lose oxygen in your blood then there is no oxygen getting to the vital organs either. That is what causes organ failure of the liver and kidney. Initially it was thought the lung complications from Covid-19 were a form of Adult Repsiratory Distress Syndrome known as ARDS. In China the early cases were thought to be some kind of atypical pneumonia. Because the virus binds to the haem part of the haemoglobin molecule the oxidative iron cannot bind. This freed iron is highly reactive against the tissues of your body. It is then free to cause all the damage in the lungs that are evidence on radiology images. It also goes to the various organs via the bloodstream to damage the liver and kidneys. The low circulating oxygen further damages these organs as well.

My analysis may turn out not to be right but in my mind it explains all the components of the disease. The similarities between Covid-19 and carbon monoxide toxicity continue. Carbon monoxide toxicity produces a high death rate especially in diabetics, those with heart disease and obesity. The symptoms of malaise, fatigue, headaches, breathlessness and dizziness are the same. It can also cause the rapid deterioration and death and the abnormal ground glass lung opacities seen on X-ray and CT scans. Does the virus increase our carbon monoxide levels or does it mimic the action of carbon monoxide?

There is a high death rate associated with the use of ventilators in Covid-29. This also fits with the picture of carbon monoxide poisoning. Low pressure ventilation seems to be associated with a better outcome and less damage to the lungs. However early oxygenation which is a relatively simple treatment seems to work in both. As mentioned previously I would recommend purchasing a small home oxygen concentrator machine.

Maybe those ethnic minority groups heavily affected by Covid-19 are those with abnormal shaped blood cells such as sickle cell disease or thalassaemias and perhaps this impacts on oxygen carrying capacity of their blood cells in the context of Covid-19? We won't have answers to these unless large retrospective studies are carried out internationally after this pandemic subsided.

How to predict death in Covid-19

Chinese Scientists have identified three biological clues in Covid-19 patients' blood samples to predict their risk of death with up to 90 per cent accuracy. They used machine learning to analyze blood samples of patients in Wuhan and identify the three biomarkers of mortality risk 10 days early.

High levels of both an enzyme associated with tissue breakdown and a protein produced during inflammation, as well as low levels of lymphocyte white blood cells, were the key predictors. Using these markers for an early diagnosis of risk of death among people with COVID-19 is vital to prioritise care for the patients who are most at risk and to try and reduce the death rate.

The three markers are : an enzyme called lactate dehydrogenase LDH, a blood marker of infection called high sensitivity C- reactive protein or hsCRP , and white blood cells in the immune system called lymphocytes. All three can be easily collected in any hospital. According to the authors this simple model can help to quickly prioritise patients, especially during a pandemic when limited healthcare resources have to be allocated.

It is reported that in Wuhan between 13.8 per cent to 19.1 per cent of COVID-19 patients became severely ill. There had been no prognostic biomarker to distinguish patients that require immediate medical attention. The researchers used a database of blood samples from 485 infected patients in the region of Wuhan between January 10th and February 18th 2020.
The researchers were able to identify the most common characteristics in the patients who had died. The accuracy of the algorithm was 90 per cent and could be applied to any blood sample taken throughout a patient's stay in hospital. This is turn can "predict" the high risk patients that need intensive early treatment when seen by a doctor.

STEP 10 HOW DO I MOVE ON WITH LIFE?

"I became the creator of myself. From the midst of darkness I became my own source of light" Cristen Rodgers

The return to the new normal: life after the pandemic. What can we learn from the aftermath of a Pandemic ? What has Covid-19 taught us? Can we go back to our normal lives and do we actually want to? How will we utilise this learning experience ? At the moment there are no treatments nor vaccine for the Coronavirus-19. Nevertheless even if there are some new options we still have the threat of further highly contagious pandemics in the future. Is this being negative or realistic? This pandemic has held a magnifying glass up to our society and focussed a spotlight on some of our ineffectual and inept leadership which in a moment of predicted crisis implemented such policies that lead to thousands of unnecessary deaths. The fact that many large "first world" countries were so unprepared and so disjointed in their major incident policies is astounding. In moments of crisis many people regress to a position of withdrawal and dependency at the cost of our civil liberties. Identity politics may again be brought to the forefront of our politics all uniting against a common "enemy" in this case China. This can bring about the unfortunate position of grasping on to known incompetent leaders in order to ease our exasperation. Only the November elections will prove whether this theory is correct or not. Perhaps one major lesson is to take back our personal control of crises in our lives by being personally prepared.

What if our country had a major nuclear or chemical attack - where was our emergency stockpile of masks and PPE?

Will we relinquish our individual rights and agree to compulsory vaccination and other treatments, tracking apps, and immunity passports? These exceptional actions may become part of our day to day lives.Our response to Covid-19 will have an immense impact on future generations. We have no choice but to recalibrate our expectations and goals.

Everything may be different in your life. Embrace the opportunity that life has given you for change and prosperity in your new existence. Be realistic and flexible - do you still want to live in a big bustling city? Will you need to pivot your work life into a new area with more demand? Utilise the lockdown period to take advantage of as many free online courses as you can manage to gain additional skills to improve your cv and portfolio.

You will need to adjust your expectations and although some of the parameters are unknown , it will give you added confidence.

Refrain from the urge to have rebound extravagance in your spending after this crisis. There may be the enticement of slipping back into bad habits again and returning to the previous spending patterns after the pandemic. You need to be proactive.

There is a lot of uncertainty in the future which may exacerbate our anxiety levels. We may be living in a world with fewer actual shops and mainly virtual interactions. Our person to person contact may be completely diminished with further social distancing and isolation. Many with mental health issues may deteriorate. But we must not dwell too much on the uncertain, unknown and uncontrollable. Maybe Covid-19 will be a catalyst to address all those urgent issues we have neglected for so long such as environmental issues, global warming, unnecessary air travel and overcrowding. Maybe society can use this as an opportunity for solidarity and unity. The main thing is not to fear the future. Use mindfulness to live in the present. This pandemic crystallises the need for living in the present even more than anything before.

When the situation is really challenging, look for ways to make life just a little bit easier and practice forgiveness for yourself and others.

Don't forget you have survived a major trauma in you and your family's lives. Be flexible with your previous high standards and grant yourself moments of comfort and relaxation.

The emotions in this stage of the pandemic will be different : creativity, skepticism, acceptance, impatience, hope, energy, and enthusiasm. You will be wholeheartedly committing to a whole new lifestyle. Harness your new found energy to increase productivity and morale. Reorient yourself to your new life. Reconnect with the world in a new way. Remember to tell your loved ones how much they mean to you and embrace all the vital things in life - compassion, kindness, health, love, family and friends. Find the silver lining- focussing on the positives in what can feel like a period of endless gloom and doom can actually help you feel better about your situation. Maybe this pandemic was a stark reminder to us of what is important to cherish in life. As the famous Native American saying goes "May the stars carry your sadness away, May the flowers fill your heart with beauty, May hope forever wipe your tears away, and may silence make you forever strong".

ABOUT THE AUTHOR

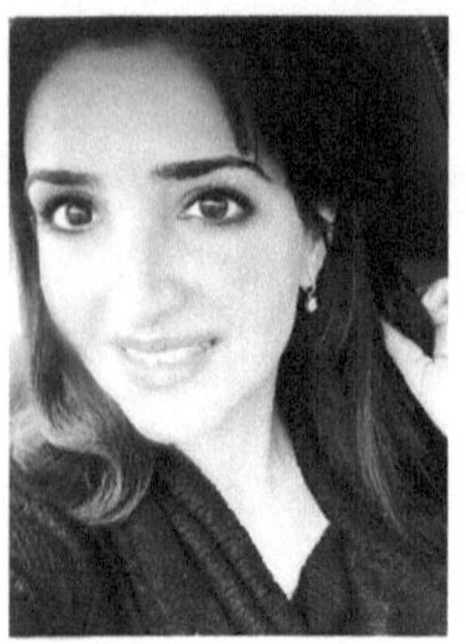

Writer, Doctor, and Surgeon Dr Megan is the author of the Little Black Book of Survival Series providing a guide to difficult situations in life. She is a full time doctor based in London, United Kingdom. She underwent her training in a number of large teaching hospitals in the United Kingdom. You can visit her online at instagram @sparklygirl_drmegan